Closure:
Surviving 3rd Degree Burns

Bianca Mya & Kendrick Turner

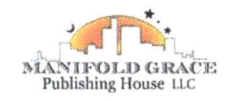

MANIFOLD GRACE
Publishing House LLC

Closure: Surviving 3rd Burns
Copyright © 2021 Bianca Mya and Kendrick Turner

All rights reserved. No part of this book may be copied or reproduced in any form without written permission from the publisher.

Cover design: Torry L. Moore
                  Jevon Saunders

ISBN: 978-1-952926-01-3

Printed in the United States of America

Published by Manifold Grace Publishing House, LLC
www.manifoldgracepublishinghouse.com
Southfield, Michigan 48033

Dedication

I dedicate this book to my 3 children:

Ka'Niyah

Ka'Nijah

Kendrick

My twin, Brittney Sherell

My sister, Brandi Stanford

My brother, Eddie Wayne Jr.

GG

Mrs. Carol Ryan

Anyone who is a burn survivor and/or a survivor of child abuse

Acknowledgments

I would like to acknowledge:
My best friend Nieja Wayns
Torry Moore
Amanda Lee
Nakayla Sheree
Gg and Papa
James Roquemore III
Audrey Roddy
Persondra Stimage
Officer AJ
Officer Dan Snyder
Children's Hospital (Columbus, Ohio)
Erica Carter (receptionist)
Dr. Rajan Thakkar
Dr. Dana
The Rehab Unit
The Burn Unit
Prosecutor Eric S.
Judge K. Phipps

Table of Contents

	Dedication	v
	Acknowledgment	vii
	Forewords	xi
	Introduction	xvii
1	BURNED!	1
2	The Kindness of Others	11
3	Rehab	17
4	Fading Scars	23
5	Heading Home	25
6	Going Viral	31
7	Closure!	37
8	Facts About Child Abuse	41
9	Block Party	43
	About the Authors	49

Forewords

I see horrible things almost every day, but it is the true nightmares that cling to my memory. I've lost track of the numbers of homicides, shootings, stabbings, rapes, beatings, and suicides I have been called to. All of them are horrible, however, there is nothing worse than when a child is the victim. I remember the faces of those suffering, but it's the screams and the wailings of their loved ones that haunt me. When a person's heart has been forever broken, when their whole world has fallen down and an ocean of suffocating grief has enveloped them, the tortured sounds of their pain can stop me dead in my tracks and fill my heart with despair. I fight this. I must remain composed and detached. I steel myself from feeling in these moments so I can think clearly. If I am calm, I can save lives. If I am collected, I can preserve the evidence that may give the victim a shred of justice. If I restore order from the terror and chaos, I can help.

Later, when it's quiet and I am alone, I reflect on what I've witnessed. I don't hide from these memories; I face them down. I try to understand what occurred and the motivations of all involved, including the emotions that created or resulted from the incident. It is then, that I allow myself to feel. I try to fathom the pain of the victims and their loved ones. My heart hurts for them. Knowing loss myself, I can relate to their suffering. I am able to dissect these tragedies, gaining a sort of perspective. I have to make peace with what I see. If I can witness the nightmares and maintain my center, I can continue to help.

When I met Bianca and KenKen, I did not know what all had occurred. I knew that Ken had been scalded by Bianca's former boyfriend and that he had to go through a significant number of surgeries to help heal his body. I promptly discovered how powerfully optimistic and charismatic Bianca is. Negativity slides by as she makes her way through life, utterly unmoved by its passing. Her unwavering dedication to her children inspires me, every day, to make myself a better father. Bianca doggedly pursues her goals in the building of her business, her charity work, or the honing of her culinary skills. Bianca's work ethic is unfaltering and tireless. She is truly an inspiration.

As I came to know the family, they entrusted me with their story, including the details of their nightmare.

In all of the quiet moments where I have sat and

dissected what I know from my semi-omniscient perspective, I can see how a hidden monster was in a position to inflict such horror, and hurt so many. Hearing about other victims of his, coming forward with their stories, I have drawn my conclusions about his creation and motivations. He is not a complicated villain in my eyes. Knowing now what he is, I understand how the events unfolded. To my mind, he was nothing more than a rattlesnake hiding in a child's crib. The snake is drawn to the warmth, but the outcome is almost inevitable.

I immediately recognize that I do not possess the frame of reference to quantify the physical pain that Ken endured. Not just at the moment of the injury, but all of the pain to follow. I pray that his young age and the passing of time block the memories from him.

When I try to envision the situation from Bianca's perspective, I am overwhelmed. I imagine how crushing her grief was when the severity of KenKen's injuries were realized; how hurt and alone she must have felt. The white-hot anger only giving way to crippling hopelessness as she was unable to comfort her child. As I reflect on her pain, that same chilling despair enters my heart with a magnitude equal to any scene I have ever experienced. I feel as though no person could endure that reality and ever be whole again. As my pondering spirals into darker levels of gloom, every time, I am interrupted with the memory of my friend's smile. Bianca's smile can brighten any room. It is beyond explanation how a person could survive such a broken heart and then become the unstoppable force of positivity and love that she is. Often Bianca will say that in the moment when she had the opportunity to exact her revenge, it was definitively God that stopped her. I will readily admit that my faith is limited, however, I can only conclude that God's will alone could have brought Bianca, KenKen and the rest of the family through that hell. It transformed them on the other side into the radiant ambassadors of love, we are blessed with today.

Officer Dan Snyder

///

One day in 2019, while perusing Facebook, a post by a Columbus Police Officer caught my attention. Spending time on social media is sometimes a waste, but in this instance, I met a wonderful young woman, and her three children! The officer was making a plea on behalf of a young woman who could use some community support moving her family, and whose youngest child had recently suffered some trauma. I knew that I could help Bianca, and probably enlist many of my friends and neighbors to do so as well.

When you first meet Bianca, she speaks quite candidly about the abuse perpetrated by a former boyfriend on her sweet baby, KenKen. And of course, as a mother, my heart bled for Ken and the girls. So, we established an early friendship, while I helped her navigate some of the issues caused by the trauma of KenKen's injuries.

Extraordinarily, what I found was not a just a woman asking for help, but an incredibly hardworking, funny, but most importantly, a parent driven to make a better life for her children.

What I have come to love and respect most about this family, is their faith and humor rising each and every day. I know that when you read this story, you'll fall in love with Bianca, Nijah, Niyah, and KenKen. It's so easy to do!

Ms. Carol Ryan

Introduction

My name is Kendrick but everyone calls me KenKen. My birthday is October 8, 2015. I was 3 years old at the time of my injuries.

I have 2 sisters, a mommy and her boyfriend; he is ok. Sometimes he's mean to me. While mommy is away, he hits me and doesn't feed me or my sisters when we are hungry. He yells at us and throws our toys away. All he does is play video games. And acts nice when mommy comes home. One day when mommy was at work, I'm in the room playing with my sisters and I poop my pants. He got mad at me, and burns my legs and my bottom in the hot water in the bathtub.

Me and mommy tell our story. Mommy helped me with my part.

1. BURNED!

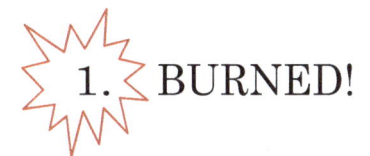

Hi my name is Kendrick but a lot of people call me KenKen. I can do some sign language and I point to the things that I want and need. This is my story.

I was 3 years old when I was hurt by a monster because I messed up my pants. The monster ran a tub of hot water and sat me in the tub. I suffered 2nd and 3rd degree burns from the waist down. As I screamed and hollered, he got me dressed to cover what he had done ... mom thought it was just my feet.

He got me dressed and held me while I pulled back the skin on my feet, until my mom came home from work.

Mommy rushed me to the hospital, crying. I didn't know why mommy was crying, so I started to cry.

They rushed me back to the burn unit and started to

cut my clothes off.

Waking up in the I.C.U., having so many medicines, hearing beeps from the machines and having tubes up my nose, I didn't know what was going on or what to think. Then again, I'm only 3 years old.

Mommy:
Looking at my baby lying in ICU I had so many mixed emotions. I felt helpless, lost, hurt and confused, as a parent. I didn't know what to think. I didn't know how I could help him. All I wanted to do was take the pain away. I even asked God why this had to happen to my family. I was so annoyed, frustrated and pissed off that this happened.

Then, patient transport keeps coming to get him at all hours of the night. I'm thinking, "Let him sleep, he's been through enough". But they have to do their job right? It's 2:00 a.m. when we get on the elevator and I am exhausted. I haven't even been to sleep.

I say, "Good morning," to patient transport, his name is Mr. Sherwin. "I'm so tired of this. Just want my kid to be better, the guy I was dating tried to kill my son!"

We began to talk and he said, "I will pray for you and

your family." And that was the last time I saw him for a while.

KenKen:
Once I left ICU, I moved upstairs to the burn unit to start my recovery. I remember being in so much pain I couldn't talk. All I could do was scream and cry. I couldn't get comfortable either. They put an artificial skin on me. I think they said it was fish skin and it will play out on its own; any areas needing skin grafts they will fix. They let me know it was going to take some time. I hated to pee or poop because it would burn so bad. It took six or seven people to change me because I would scream and jump around from the pain. Days went by and I'm still so miserable and in pain. It didn't seem like nothing could take this pain away, but mommy lying next to me in bed.

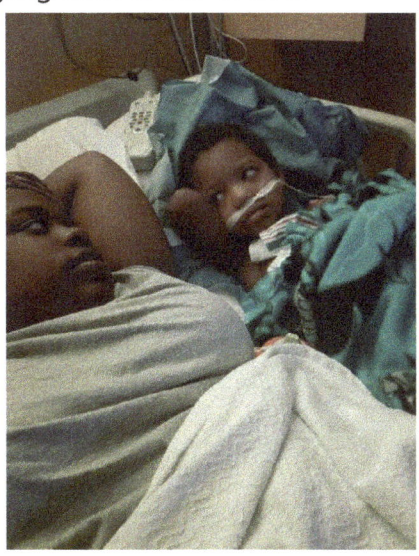

I'm thinking, being out of ICU is such a big relief, now we can start the road to recovery. And my girls, Nijah and Niyah, can come to visit now. Ken still has to have surgeries and be sedated according to the doctors. Whenever he would pee or poop - he would scream in pain. Sometimes I would leave out of the room because I just couldn't look at him looking at me for help. This was something I couldn't help with. As a parent, watching your child suffer and you can't help, is the worst thing ever. Days went by and it seems like KenKen was getting better. I'm thinking, we've got a long road here. Ken's doctor's name was Rajan Thakkar, he tells us we're going to be here for a while - at least a couple of months. Days and weeks went by. Seems like it's taking forever for the healing to start.

Then the news wants me to share my story, so I have an interview with "6 On Your Side" news to tell what happened. Maybe it will shed some light on child abuse. What's the worst that could happen? So Rich, from the church, came over and we walked across the street to Panera Bread so I could share my story. I had met Richard and his step-son, Jimmy, a few months back at the family shelter. That's where we were until we got a place of our own.

The "It Takes a Village" segment of the news aired my story the same night. My phone is suddenly ringing off the hook! The next day Ken felt like a kid in a candy store. So many balloons, teddy bears, stuffed animals and toys began to fill the room. Here I was, wondering what was next and we start to receive love mail and best wishes. It was so much so, to the point doctors and nurses would walk past the room then come back and say, "Wow, in all the years I've been here, I've never seen a room like this. This little boy is loved." And, "Hey, this reminds me of the movie UP! Wow, where is all this coming from?"

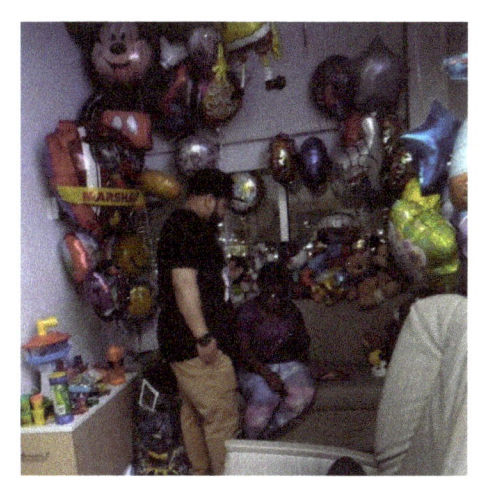

Gifts for KenKen

People were telling me, "We saw you on the news last night, we are praying for you." "We love you and KenKen and admire your strength." Even the nurses would say, "We commend you for leaving him!" I was confused, "Why wouldn't I leave him?" They explained, "We see so many moms stay with the guy that hurts the kids." I can't even believe it, just shaking my head.

Hearing these things made me feel a lot better. It made me feel loved to know that my little boy is so loved. His room filled with so much love, and the prayers really helped Ken's recovery, gave him a speedy healing. I'm so grateful for the many, many people who sent best wishes, love, prayers, thoughts, and concerns. They truly made a difference in me and Ken's life. The kindness of strangers is what really helped us push through. People from all over the map reached out, prayed, and lent a hand, real support.

KenKen:
I started getting love mail, stuffed animals, balloons and toys. I found a new love for superheroes. People would send any superhero to make me feel better and to my surprise, it did help. Whenever I came out of surgery, I would identify some of the new things in the room. The balloons and stuffed animals made me smile I begin to pull on the balloons and play with them. I started to play with my superheroes and I would put on my batman cape. The nurses started to call me Super Ken and that made me smile. I have my own name now; Super Ken is what they call me.

I'm starting to feel like myself just a little bit. I'm starting to move around more and stand on my own.

The surgeries are going well. Physical therapy helps a lot.

Mommy:
With so much love in the room Ken started to get out of bed to be pushed around the hallway in his wheelchair. Not long after, he would begin physical therapy. He would learn to hate it because they made him work. He would get out of his bed and sit on a mat where he had to learn to lay on his stomach to have tummy time and stretch the new skin on the front of his body. His sisters would come and lay on the floor and play superheroes with him. That really helped.

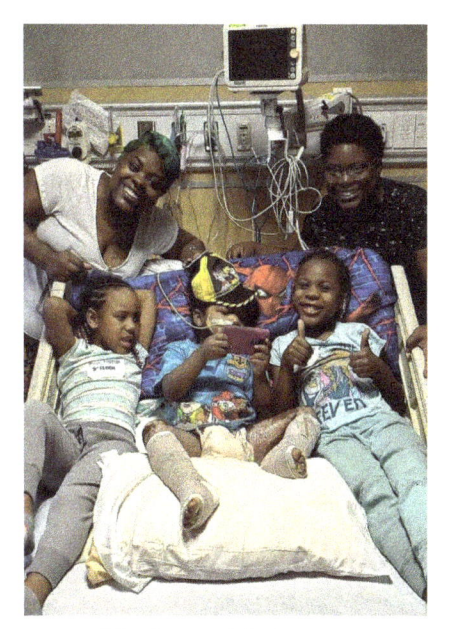

Playing with Ken

Ken was slowly coming back to himself, laughing and playing, wanting to get into the wheelchair and be pushed around.

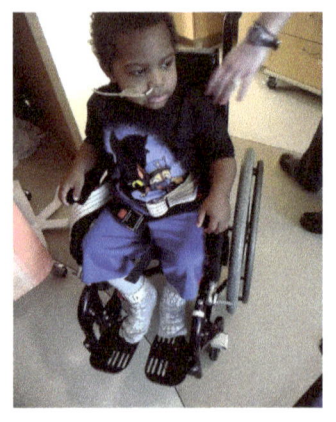

Ken started getting out of bed to be on the mat. He had leg braces that he needed to wear whenever he was in bed or moving around. But whenever he had visitors, Ken would try to stand up with the braces on, still not strong enough to stand on his own. He had the determination, will power and super hero strength to stand up and to keep going.

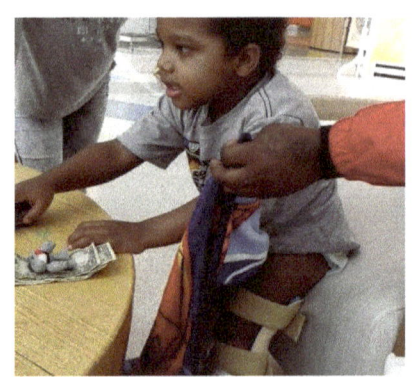

New leg braces for Super Ken

"Prayer works!" There's "power in prayer." KenKen is healing so well! He's moving more, he's standing on his own. He even wants to get out of bed on his own. This is amazing. The doctors are also as amazed at his recovery and progress. Although he is moving around, he still needs surgery; a skin graph because his skin isn't healing as it should. So, they scheduled surgery for two days out. The night before surgery, KenKen catches the flu. I'm thinking, OMG, then I remember what the reporter, her name was Mandy, said. "Don't get upset, this may be a blessing in disguise," which it was. They checked Ken, changed his dressing and came back saying, "Kendrick's right foot is completely closed, he only needs a graft on one foot but if it closes before the next scheduled surgery, he won't need the graft." I am at a loss for words right now. "God, I see you out here working for us!"

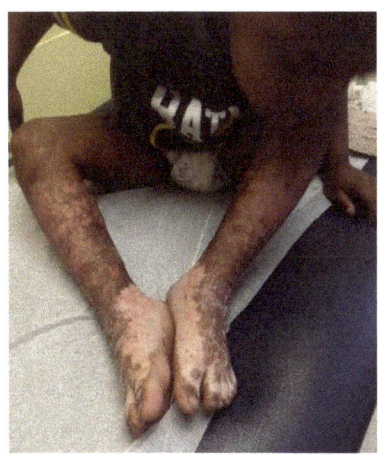

Ken checking out his legs and feet

2. The Kindness of Others

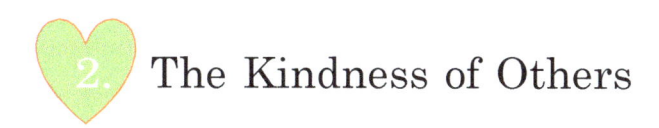

The kindness of strangers helped get me through
When I was lost, felt like stuck in glue
There were so many of you to see me through
Walk me thru and talk me thru
And for that I'm grateful for you - so many of you
The kindness of others brought me through dark days And into the light
The kindness of others helped me…

TT (auntie) Brittney flew in from Atlanta to be my support person because Lia couldn't stay. So, Lia would just come up during the day. Now I have my twin Brittney, my friend Nakayla, Ms. Audrene and Richard. These four were heaven sent, they haven't missed a beat. They've been right by my side with tears and love. Lia was my old general manager at my job. We became real close during the years we worked together. Kayla, I met Nakayla at the shelter too. She has two girls and one boy like me, so we were really close and helped each other out a lot. Kayla kept the girls the two months I sat in the hospital with KenKen, and TT Mary would get them sometimes. Ms. Audrene was like the momma of the workplace at the airport, always cleaning and decorating and praying for you if you needed it. The sweetest lady I've ever met. Richard and Audrene came up every day, didn't miss a beat. I'm thinking, this is what love has got to be. I am truly surrounded by love.

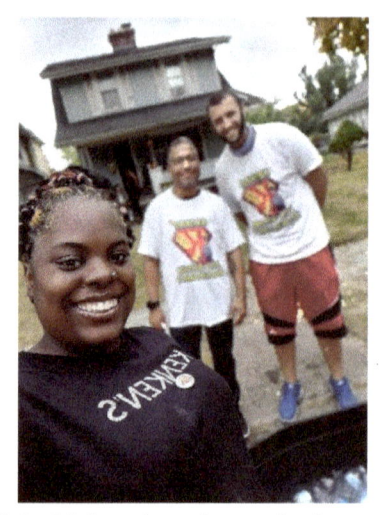

With Richard and son-in-law,
Mr. Jimmy

This helped me keep my mind right, although I'm missing my girls. They would come up after school and go to the clubhouse. Clubhouse was like therapy for kids of the sick patient, which was really needed because Niyah needed help. Niyah was my 6-year-old who, at the time, witnessed Ken get hurt. She even tried to get him out of the tub. Can you picture that? Breaks my heart. Niyah is having trouble in school.

Nijah is an emotional wreck. Her teacher took another job out state; all of this on top of her baby brother being hurt. How much can a 6-year-old take? The school is across the street from the hospital but I can't, and don't wanna leave KenKen. TT Brittney, TT Brandi, Ka'Nijah my big sister, Papa and GG tried their best to work with Niyah. But Niyah is completely out of it. She had spells where she had to be admitted to the hospital. So, now I got a kid in the burn unit and one in the psych ward. Lord, this can't be my life right now. Lord what is it that you need me to do? I've been nothing but patient since day one. I kept being still and patient and God sent so many blessings my way, I can't even count. I truly appreciate those who have been placed into our lives.

Ms. Viola called to set up an appointment to come back to the house and start early learning for KenKen. I had met her a week prior to Ken getting hurt. I explained to her what happened and she said ok, no worries. The next day Ms. Viola showed up at the hospital and said, "Don't worry about schooling, I'm here for you." She came up once a week as if we were at home. She sat in the room and talked with me and Brittney. She even went to the operating room a few times (If this ain't support then I don't know what is!). She was there as a mom, a friend, an auntie. She was there like family.

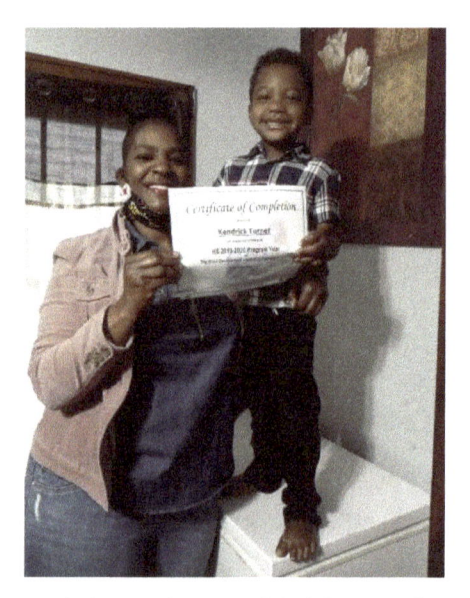

Ms. Viola and Ken with his certificate

A few coworkers stopped by, even the station manager, Rey, came by. Thank you Mark, Corey, and Kyla. Big thanks you to GAT (Ground Airline Transportation, we service American Airlines.

My job told me to take as much time as I needed and not to worry, my job would be here when I was ready. My landlord was more than cool, he would send a text here and there, checking on us, and he lives in

Washington state. That was pretty cool.

Persondra and Jonesha drove down from Port Huron, Michigan, spent the weekend with us. TT Brittney and Jonesha took the girls swimming at the hotel so that gave Brittney a break away from the hospital. I got to get some rest while she was here. She would sometimes fuss at the nurses because she thought they were hurting Ken. But nope, just doing their jobs.

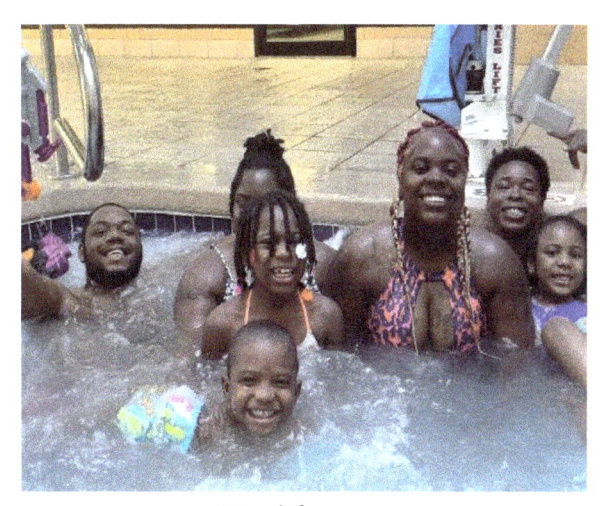

Pool fun

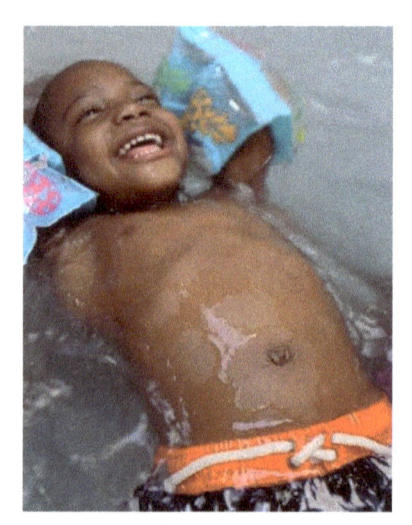

Pool therapy

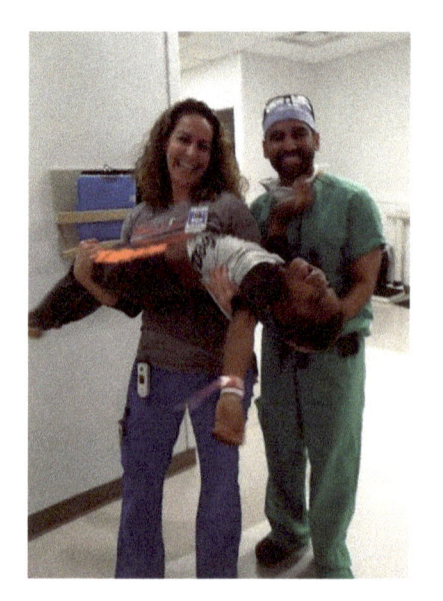

Dr. Rajan Thakkar and nurse

3. Rehab

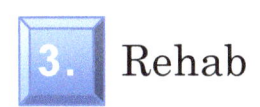

Back to KenKen's recovery - one night Ken snatched the IV out of his arm, so they had to take him down to put it back in. Now he has to wear arm restraints so it doesn't keep happening.

No skin grafts were needed so we were moved to the 9th floor, to rehab. Rehab means we should be closer to going home right? We did not know it was going to be a tough rehab. Every day we were put on a set schedule of working out - every day. That means Kendrick is going to have to get up and be active.

The first day in rehab: 8a.m. wake up. Kendrick is put on a walker and walking the halls. He's able to move his legs, so his legs no longer need to be elevated. That means he gets a new wheelchair. The first day Ken got his wheelchair, he takes off like a pro (kids adapt quick and easy).

Now, Kendrick meets a friend, Harper Grace. Harper has been in the hospital since January 10th. He knows she has a rare condition called acute flaccid myelitis. If you don't know what that is, it is also known as AFM. AFM is a virus that causes fever and respiratory symptoms. Harper had it worse, at only 5 years old she had to be in a wheelchair and learn to walk again, kinda like KenKen. Harper was in the room right next to his. They became friends and would sometimes do therapy together and race their wheel chairs together down the hall. They would paint together. I met Harper's mom, Ashley, and we became friends.

Ashley and I would chit chat about what happened to our kids. She is pregnant with another little girl, Tensile. I can imagine how she is feeling being pregnant. I have two other kids, so I understand. Everyone loved Harper and Ken, they were so fun together.

Kendrick is kicking butt in rehab. Now we just need him to EAT, so his feeding tube can be taken out. One issue is, KenKen doesn't have an appetite so TT Brandi, TT Brittney and one of the nurses would have a race to see who could eat the most Gogurts and fruits and Kendrick would always win. This was good. It counted as nutrients for him. Nana Audrey came to see us from Port Huron, Michigan because our mom is her daughter and we are her grandkids and greatgrand

-kids. We love Nana! (This is what Nana tells the kids whenever she talks to them) She brought us all types of goodies and snacks and she is fun, she painted pictures with us.

I walked downstairs with my twin sister and felt like I was in a new world. I hadn't left the hospital in like a month and a half. I barely came out of the room. I remember standing at the information desk talking to Ms. Tanya and the other lady who sat there. They would ask how's everything? Brittney had obviously made some friends, because I don't know any of these people, and I wonder how they know what's going on.

While standing at the desk I saw Mr. Sherwin. He came over and asked how I was doing. I said I was blessed and better than the last time we talked. Brittney walked over and he looked amazed. He said, "Wait, it's two of y'all?"
I said, "Yeah!"
He asked, "So which one of y'all have I been talking to?"
Brittney says, "Me".
He said, "Wwowwwwww!"
Brittney said to me, "This is the one I was telling you about. He wants us to come to his church and meet his wife. (Remember I met him earlier in the book? He was patient transport.

On Sunday we went to church with Mr. Sherwin who is pastor of True Love Ministries and his wife is the First Lady. Brittney and I were blown away. So, this whole time Mr. Sherwin is a pastor. He carried himself well and differently. He prayed for KenKen, talked about him at service, and that was that. We met his daughters and wife. They all worked at Children's Hospital, what a blessing! First Lady came to visit Ken in rehab and brought him some things. She even offered to help care for him once we were home from the hospital.

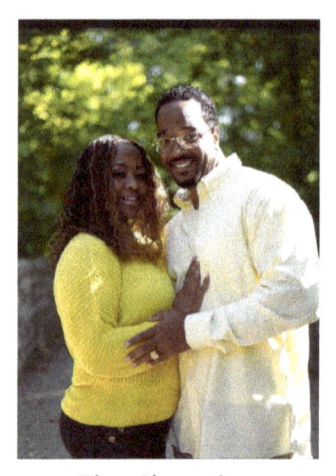

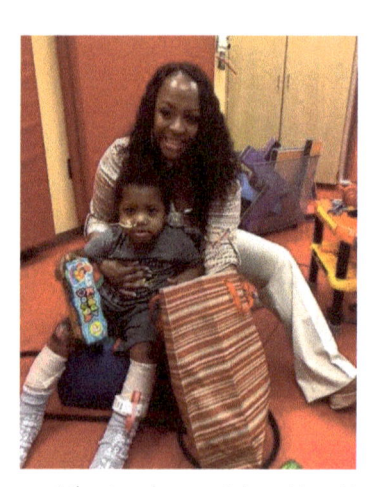

The Sherwins   1st Lady with KenKen

Ken is now ready to learn to walk again and is using a walker, but when he walks, his feet turn outward, like a penguin almost. As he walks, doctors inform me that when the skin comes back, it is tight and non-moveable. The more he moves around, the better it will get. It will loosen up. Ken is really moving and adapting well. Now he's walking up and down the stairs with help. This is so cool.

The nurses told me I need to start taking some things home soon, so it won't be so much when we leave. (This means we are closer to going home!) Ken is doing really well. A few minor setbacks though, but that's part of recovery. When we were able to go home, we sent all the balloons to the kids in the cancer ward.

They want me to begin bathing Ken and wrapping his bandages, but I don't think I'm ready. I'm thinking, they are moving too fast. He screams whenever he is near water, he is traumatized. I'm not putting him in the tub! He will get sponge baths. I feel like it's too soon for him to get back in the tub.

4. Faded Scars

I'm scarred up because of the hands of a monster
Maybe even a silent enemy
Secret hate and animosity
Wondering why someone would envy me?
I'm only three
Can't even count to three
  this man hated me
  he burned my feet
From right up underneath me
Now I can't stand to be bound by a walker and
  wheelchair
In my heart I know this is only temporary
Lord help me, I'm only three
Lord take this pain away
Help my scars to fade
Lord please fade these scars away
I'm only three
Pain medication, ICU, I'm only three
What could I have done to thee?
Mommy can't you see?
I'm crying out for you and me
Lord fade these scars away
Please heal my legs and feet
And fade these scars away
Physical therapy and moms love

My scars begin to fade away
Fading scars
My scars fade away
Fading scars

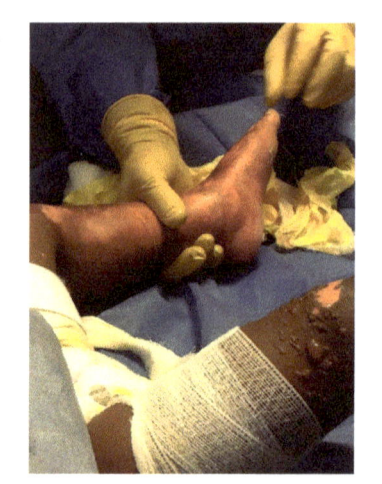

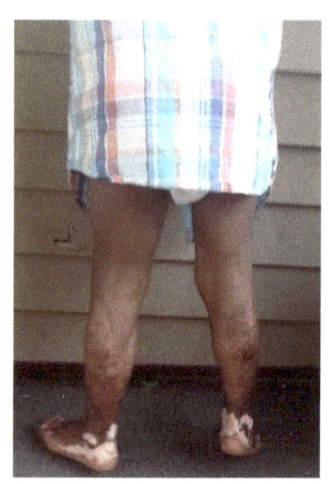

Scars are proof that you're stronger than what tried to kill you.

5. Heading Home

Tomorrow we get to be released from the hospital. So many mixed emotions about being back home. I haven't been home in two months. I've been at the hospital with Ken since the incident. I can only imagine how he feels. Ken didn't want to go into the house when we finally made it home. The last time we were there he was hurt. They sent a nurse to assist me with bandages and changes 3 times a week. Kendrick was getting bandages delivered twice a week. I'm thinking, this is crazy! How am I going to manage three kids on my own? Especially when two out of the three, needs one on one attention.

KenKen:
I'm scooting across the floor playing with toys. Our big cousin, Nuke, comes by to check on us now that we are home. Mom is spending time with the girls; I have therapy and outpatient appointments four times a week. My sister Niyah is having more trouble. Richard

and Jimmy come by often to see me and to help mommy out. I had an allergic reaction to the Neosporin and had really bad blisters on my feet. I couldn't stand up. I'm still wrapped up to my knees, I thought being home would be easier! But mommy never loses faith or seems to be frustrated.

Mommy:
Niyah Takes Flight ~ Flying Niyah to Atlanta, Georgia with TT Brittney because I can't manage KenKen and Niyah. I need help. I'm thinking of moving to Atlanta. Niyah spends time with Auntie Brittney who has to admit Niyah into the hospital. Niyah is too much for anyone to handle after seeing Ken get held down in the bathtub and trying to help him get out of the tub. It really did a number on her. She was diagnosed with disruptive behavior disorder and something with severe depression. She was badly traumatized and spent a month in the children's psych ward. They put her on three medications that I thought made her seem worse. I don't believe in medications for your feelings. Feelings and emotions change, and since I'm not going to feel like this forever, I'm not taking any meds!

She's back ~ Niyah is back and you can tell she misses her sister and now things seem to be ok. It's another holiday so we leave for the grocery store and come home to BBQ and the 4th of July. Ken and the girls are playing in the sprinkler. He has on his new colorful pressure socks, playing in the sprinkler. It's good to see them playing. Someone tried to break into my car. I call the police, they come out.

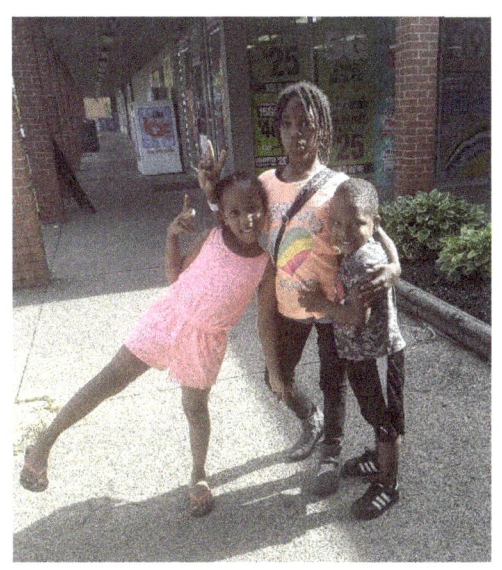

My babies, Niyah, Nijah and KenKen

They asked what was on Ken's feet and why. I explained what happened to him. I remember one officer, his name was AJ, was in the passenger seat. He said, "Wow girl, you giving me chills. I want you to follow me on social media, I have a pretty big platform. My partner and I want to come back in a week so you can share your story with the world." I'm thinking, "Yeah, whatever...just take the police report and go on."

I told them I wanted to move; you can't heal in turmoil. "We gotta get outta this house!" His partner, Office Hale got out of the car and said a prayer for me and the kids. Wow, these are some kind of officers doing this for me.

The following week Officer AJ and Officer Hale came back and did what they said they would. I had no idea who this officer was, but he is pretty well known around the city of Columbus and across the world. Long story short they moved us into our new home and I met so many people. I met a lady named Carol Ryan, you will hear more about her later in the story.

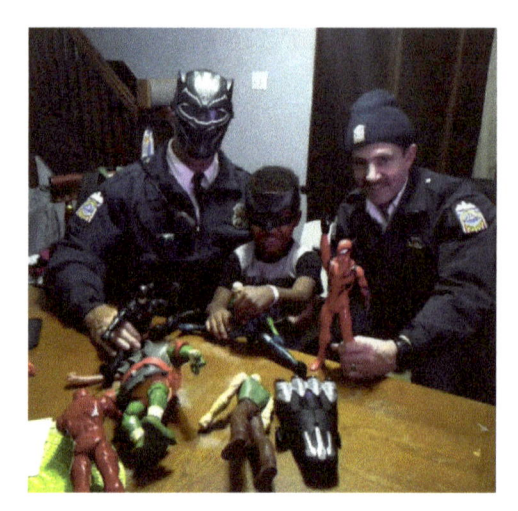

A house full of Super Heroes!

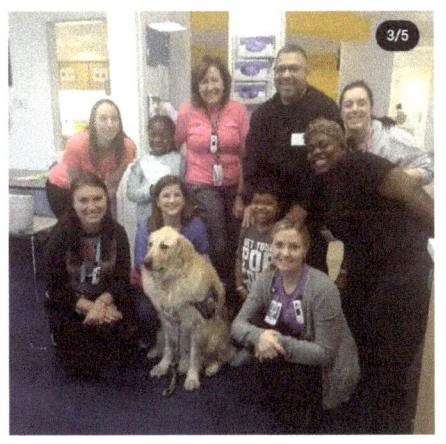

Ken's 'graduation' with Richard and staff at Rehab Center

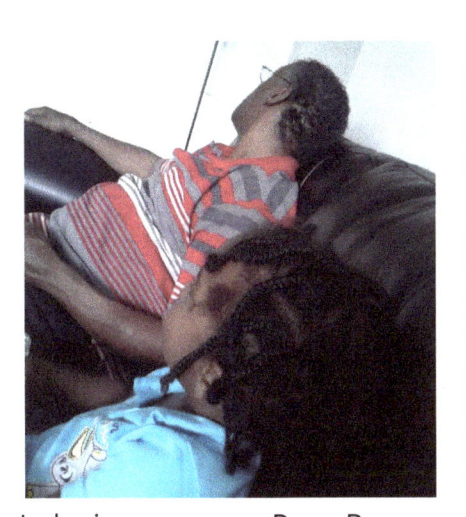

In loving memory, Papa Ron Lane passed away the day we left rehab.

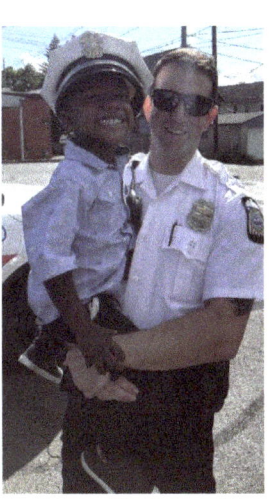

With Officer Hale

6. Going Viral

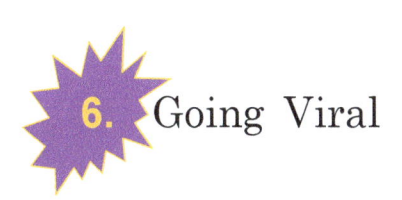

The first time we went viral was to expose Jamie for what he did to KenKen.

This time around it is because I met this cop, Officer AJ. He and other people seemed to admire our story. Or, they said I inspired them with my response to the whole situation. Had I reacted how most people would have; I'd be sitting in jail. Would've lost my kids and been all types of jacked up. Instead, I chose peace and God's comfort. God has carried me along the way and blessed me with all kinds of people. He blessed me because of my faithfulness, just trusting that everything was going be ok with KenKen. Because of Officer AJ and his partner, we are moving. AJ's precinct even raised the rest of the money I needed for the deposit on the new place.

Ms. Carol Ryan reached out and asked what was needed, then, supplied all that was needed. From couches, to dining room tables, to patio furniture, to dishes, pots and pans, I can't thank her and her friends enough. They went above and beyond expectations for me and the kids, with school supplies, clothes and shoes. This can't be my life right now, overwhelmed with thoughtfulness and love. My cup was overflowing.

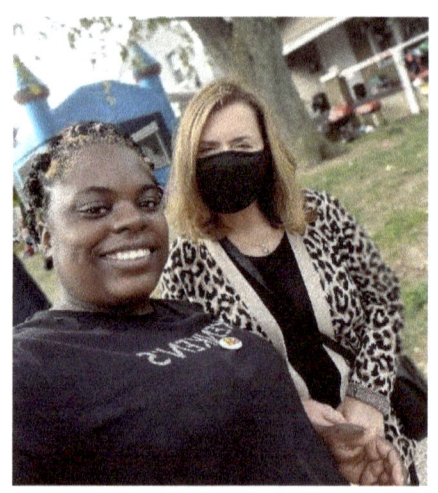

Me and Ms. Carol Ryan at the block party. She helped us make our new house a home and her husband (a dentist) takes care of the children's teeth.

Brittney and I took a trip to Lowes to see about some things for Ken so he would begin to shower and bathe again. At Lowes, we met Ms. Dawn and shared our story with her. She said she would see what she could do. Twenty-four hours later Ms. Dawn emailed Brittney saying they had a tub, sink and toilet for us - brand new. The store wanted to give it to us, along with paint and whatever else we needed to help with Ken's recovery. At the new house I painted the bathroom in Sponge Bob yellow (that was Ken's comfort zone in the hospital).

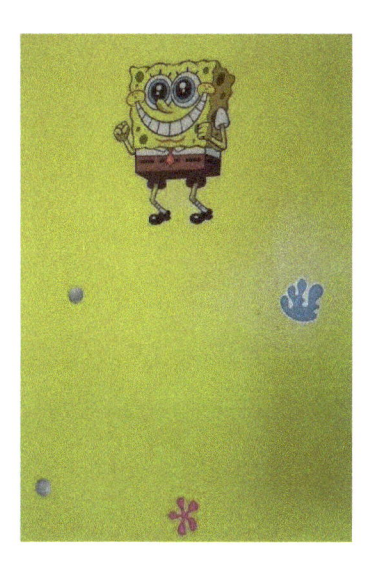

We hoped this would help him be more comfortable while using the bathroom. It helped; Ken is now potty trained. He takes a bath - with the water running. It's progress, so I'm okay with that. Things seem to be finally working out for us. Ken and the girls have met the neighborhood kids. Sara Elizabeth (neighbor) has a trampoline in her backyard that the kids play on. And Ken tags right along like he isn't bandaged up. I love it! Kids adapt very easily.

Ms. Carol is back, checking on me and the kids. My

heart is grateful for this woman who had never known me a day in her life, but is right here for me, like she knew me her whole life. Ms. Carol you are more than appreciated. Don't know how to ever thank you or repay you.

Ready for school ~ School is starting. The girls and Ken are ready. Thank you, Ms. Becky, for the school clothes. The girls are going back to the same school. KenKen is taking the bus to school. He seems to like it so far. So that's cool!

The girls are happy about the new home and about Ken being home. Niyah is getting better, not having as many breakdowns like before. So that's cool.

Ready for Ken's birthday ~ KenKen is turning FOUR! We've got to do it big for him and show appreciation to those who have been standing by us. So, I'm going to make Ken's birthday a child abuse awareness birthday block party for anybody who wants to come. It's the only way I know how to give back and say thank you and we love you. Everyone showed up and we had a great time.

Officer AJ even came by on his off day with a few officers. They raced and played games with the kids and it was a good time.

Ken is really progressing! We don't need physical therapy as much now. The burn clinic is once a month now, so we are doing well. I have depression spells and breakdowns, but I assume that's normal given the circumstances. So, I won't complain too much. Then again, I'm surrounded by so much love I can't be upset.

The winter holidays are approaching, still so loved by so many people I have nothing to worry about. Officer AJ came by with another one of his co-workers. His name is Officer Snyder. He heard about KenKen and wanted to meet us and give us tickets to Zoo Lights, that was cool, we had never been. Officer Snyder seemed pretty cool so I told him to stop by and see us sometimes. And that he did. He brought his partner, Officer Mottinger. Seems like they came over every day to say hey, or to get something that 'Mom' (me) was cooking in the kitchen.

Officer Snyder loves to eat, his favorite is mom's cookies and cream cheesecake. Pretty cool to have officers come over for something positive. So now, we have four police friends that come by to see us!

7. Closure!

Jamie was arrested in Michigan and brought back to Ohio where he would sit in jail until the trial. Or, he could take a plea, whichever comes first. I am excited about the arrest. Didn't think it would ever happen, but because of Officer Sumner and his partner Rodney Cooper in Flint, Michigan there was a quick and easy arrest. Now I can sleep a little better. It took a little over a year and a half to go to trial.

The prosecuting attorney on the case was amazing and the judge was very sweet and understanding. I read my victim impact statement:

"To whom this may concern, I am not happy with the outcome as my son, who is now 5, has suffered enough and had a crazy amount of physical and mental damage to his little body. My girls suffered emotionally and mentally and I guess you can pretty much imagine me as a mom and how I'm feeling. KenKen, who the world has grown to

love through this incident, has permanent damage to his feet. He is sometimes ashamed to show his feet because of the scars and as a mom, it hurts. He is now able to talk and asks me why he got burned (crazy right?) and I have no answer for him. But writing this letter today means we get some kind of closure and I'm ok with that, knowing that some type of justice is being served. I'm ok with it.

God Bless"

So, for me this is closure! I can feel relieved. Judge says that was the best victim statement she ever heard and that I touched her heart. And if it wasn't for covid she would have come and given me hug. I thought that was dope.

He took a plea, and only got four years. I'm ok with that, it's something. And something is better than nothing. Now I can breathe, and I am relieved.

I know I have an acknowledgement page, but I want to say THANK YOU from the bottom of my heart to so many people. I want to especially highlight my twin sister Brittney, Nieja Wayns my special friend, James Roquemore lll, Carol Ryan, Becky Defiansto, Kim Byles, Leonda Miller, Audrey Roddy, Lia Scriven, Jimmy Lewis, Richard Juarez (and family), Teal Marchande and

Nickelodeon, Officer Dan Snyder, Officer Alex Mottinger, Officer Anthony Johnson (AJ), Officer Curtis Hale (and his wife), Officer Amanda Hoover, Sergeant James Fuqua, Sergeant Rashawn Sykes, Officer Sumner and his partner Rodney Cooper (of Flint, Michigan) and many more. You all hold a special place in my heart for the love and kindness you have for, not only me and my children, but other people too. You all are appreciated and loved more than you know. And this is the only way I know to say thank you. You all have played major roles in my life since meeting you in 2019. And you all continue to be here for me and my babies, you have brought me out of dark times in the smallest ways whether it was a drop in or stopping by. Maybe it was a card, a gift, a call, or text.

Can't do much to repay you, except acknowledging you all through this book. If I did not mention your name, please blame my head and not my heart. I love you and thank you!

Big thank you to Ms. Darlene for being patient with me through the process of this book. I've started and stopped many times and you waited patiently. Thank you and I love you.

8. Facts About Child Abuse

1. 1 in 7 children in the U.S. has experienced child abuse, and/or neglect.
2. Neglect is the most common form of child abuse.
3. In 2018, 76% of child abuse perpetrators were a parent to their victim.
4. Children who experience any form of violence in childhood have a 13% greater chance they will not graduate high school.
5. Child abuse hotline, 24/7 at 1.800.422.4453

9. Block Party

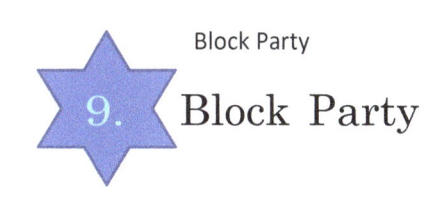

Every year we give a block party for KenKen's birthday and to raise awareness about child abuse. The community is invited and we provide food, fun and games along with information about child abuse. The t-shirts, caps and other items raise money to fund the party. Here are pictures of the block party and KenKen's journey!

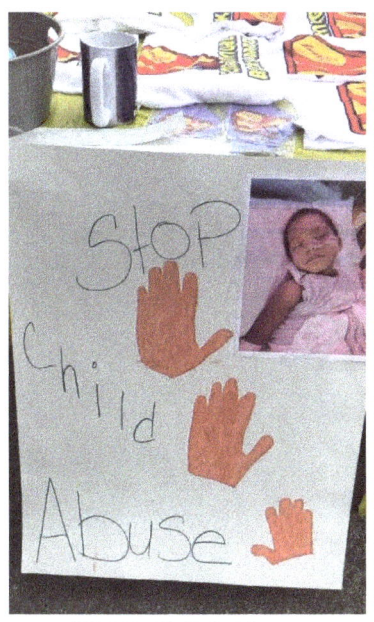

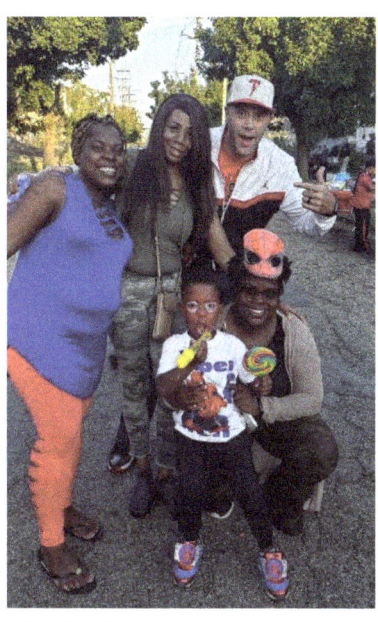

STOP Child Abuse   Ms Andrea, AJ and Brittney

Closure: Surviving 3rd Degree Burns

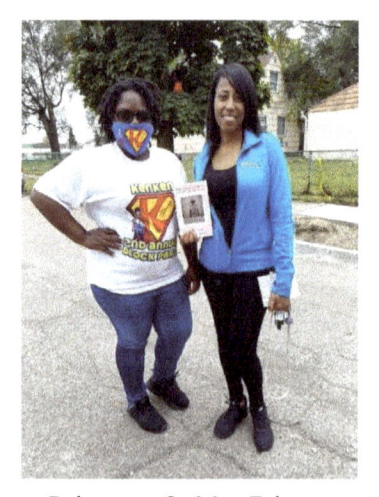

Brittney & Ms. Erica

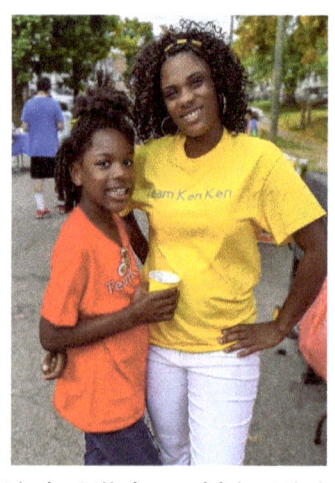

Little Nijah and big Nieja

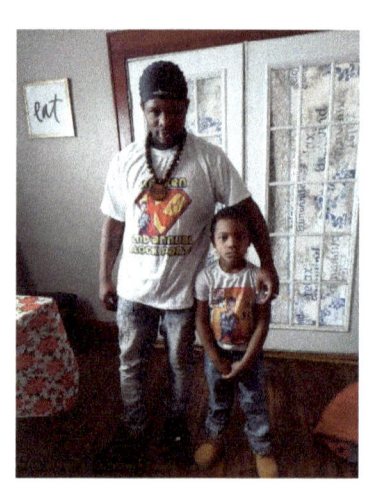

Video game partners, James

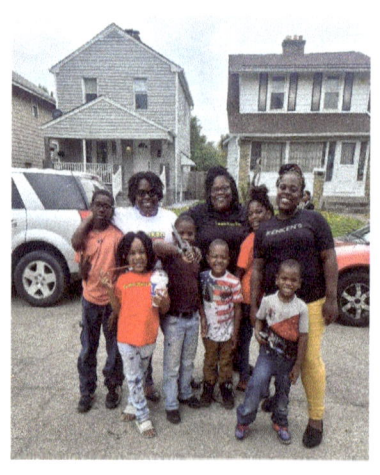

The gang

44

Block Party

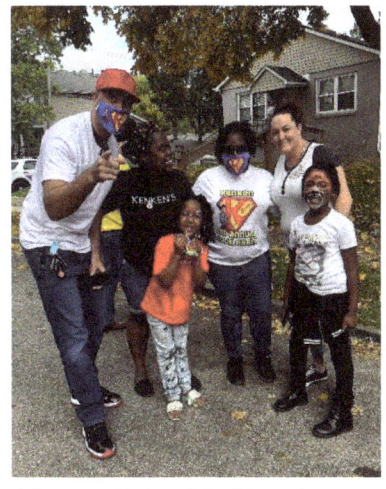

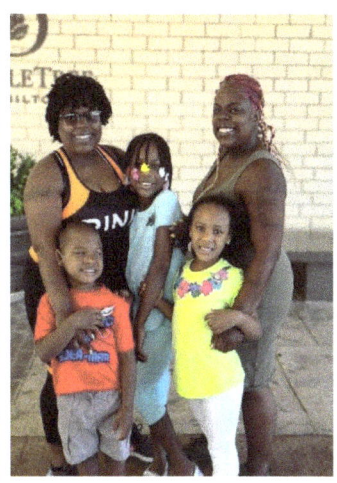

AJ, me, Britt, Ms Heather   Mi familia

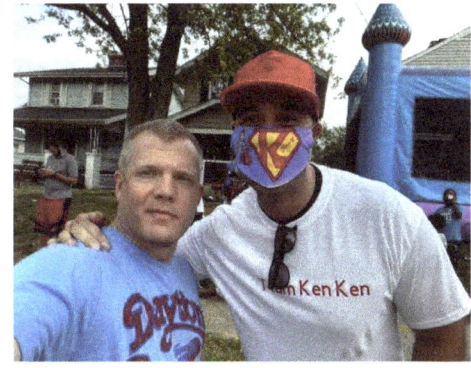

Bill and Officer AJ

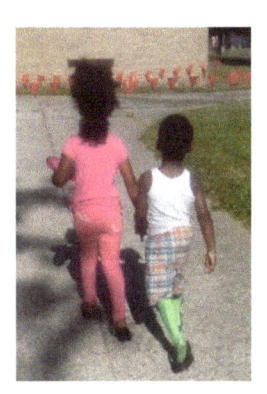

Summer school & compression socks

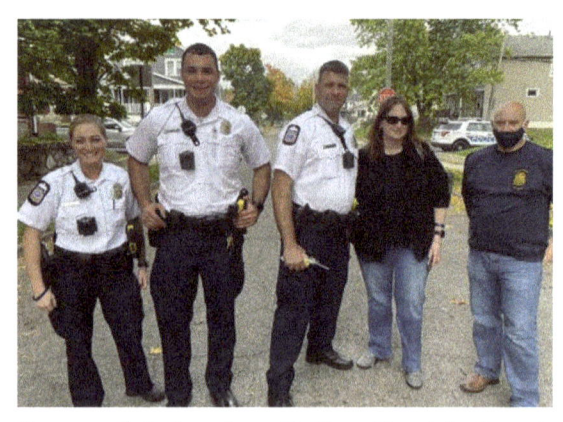

Some of Columbus Police Dept.'s finest: Officers Amanda Hoover, Dan Snyder, Alex Mottinger, Nicole Starfish, former Deputy Chief

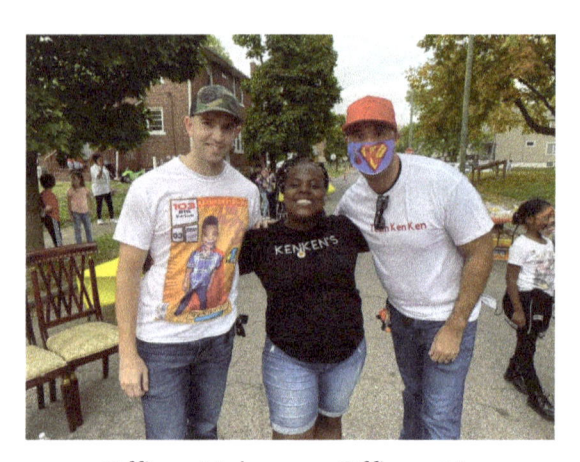

Officer Hale, me, Officer AJ

Block Party

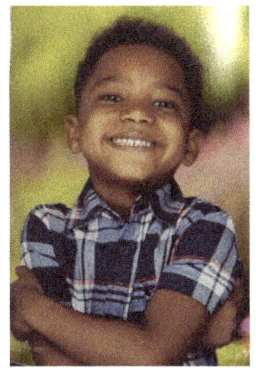

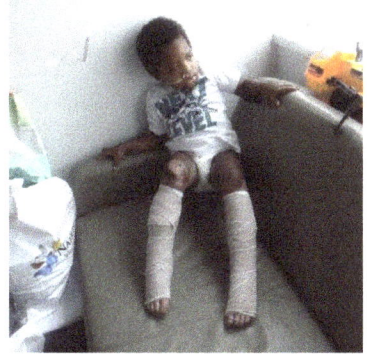

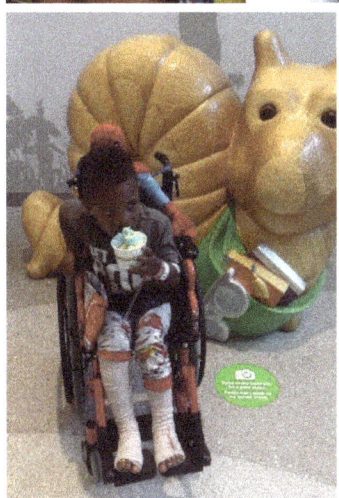

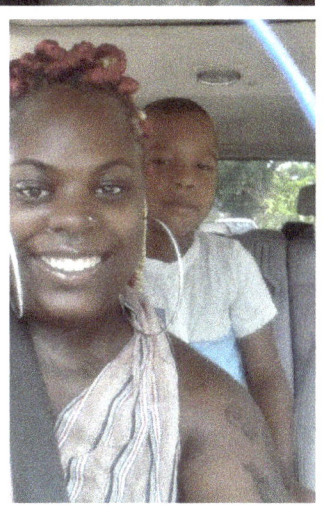

Ice cream after surgery

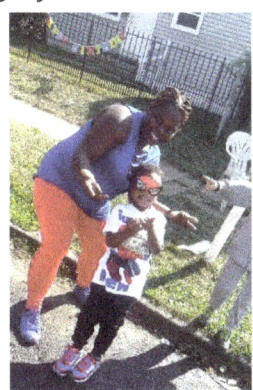

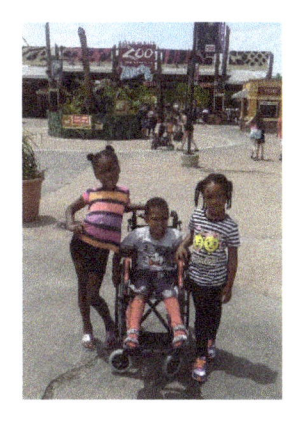

Closure: Surviving 3rd Degree Burns

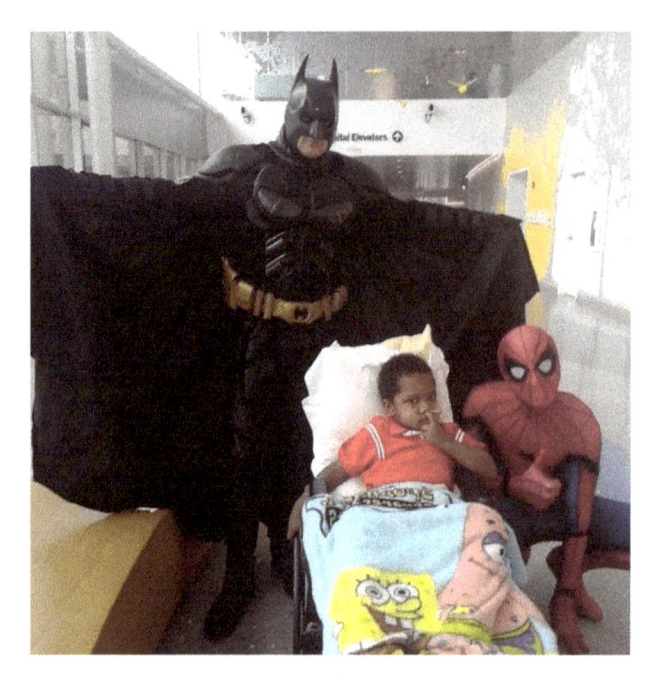

Special Visitors

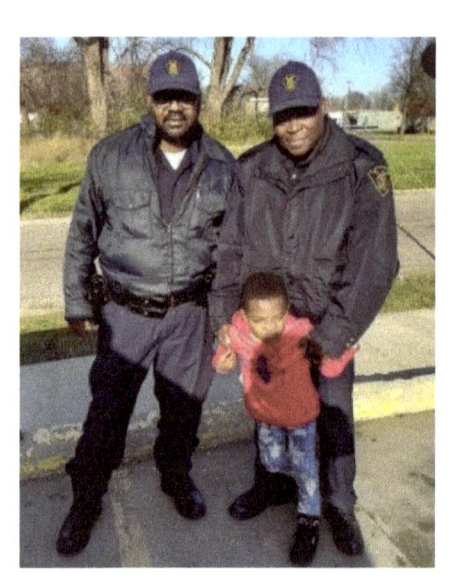

MSP, Ronnie Sumners & Rodney Cooper of Flint with Ken. They caught the monster.

About the Authors

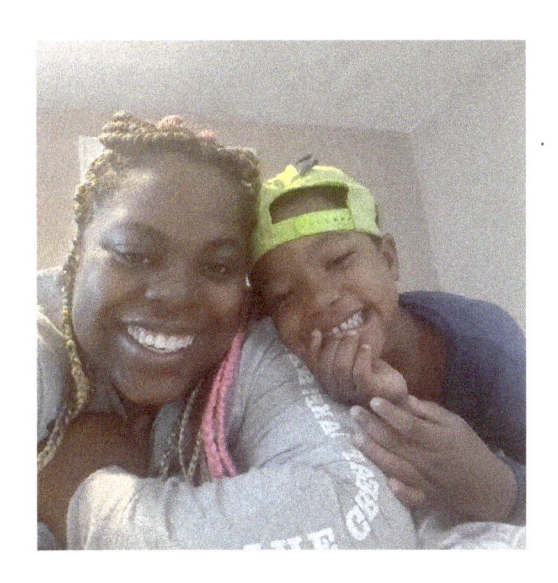

Bianca Mya was born in Flint, Michigan on March 24, 1992 (one of two), yes, a twin. She was adopted at the age of 12 and graduated from Port Huron High School. Bianca has a license in Culinary Arts and loves cooking for her family and friends. She has worked at John Glenn International Airport for the last 7 years. Bianca is something of a phenomenon in her community. She is a person who has been through so much, yet she gives even more. Bianca loves her community and tries to incorporate love and peace in everything she does. She brings those together who are different in every walk of life to coexist as one.

Bianca has the most amazing faith-based outlook on life. God's love shines through her in every act of kindness from feeding those around her, taking people into her home, and building them up. To the most extreme acts of showing those around her no matter what is thrown your way, God's plan for you is always bigger. Bianca plans to reach lives and touch their spirit with her story and how she overcame and loved beyond the pain. The world is so much better with people like Bianca who can bring everyone together and show it's ok to not be ok at times.

KenKen

This would not be a story without Ken. At this writing he is 5 years old and is healing nicely. Unfortunately, he is healing in the corona pandemic and like millions of kids around the world doesn't get to run, jump and play with other kids like before. But he is a strong little boy and a hero to many. Permanent scars? Flashbacks? This little boy, despite this terrible thing that happened to him, has experienced so much love and worked so to get better, flashbacks will only remind him that with God he can overcome anything! #KenKenstrong

About the Authors

To keep up with KenKen's journey or contact Bianca:

Instagram: iamkenken5
Website: www.kenkenstrong.com
Email: kendrickandmommy@gmail.com